ESSENTIAL GUIDE TO VITILIGO

Understanding, Managing, and Thriving with Vitiligo: An In-Depth Exploration in the Essential Guide to Skin Health

DR. CASEY LOREN

DISCLAIMER

This book's content is only meant to be used for general informative purposes. Although the author has taken great care to ensure the content is accurate and thorough, no warranties or assurances on the information's accuracy, correctness, or reliability are provided. It is recommended that readers employ their own judgment and discretion when applying any material found in this book to their particular situation.

The information in this book is not intended to replace professional advice, nor is the author an expert in any of the subjects covered. It is recommended that readers consult with experienced professionals regarding any particular issues or concerns.

Any name that may be mentioned or referred in this book does not imply endorsement, recommendation, or relationship on the part of the author with any person, entity, good, website, or association. These references are made only for informational purposes and are not meant to be taken as recommendations or endorsements.

The information contained in this book may cause readers to suffer loss or damage, for which the author disclaims all obligation and accountability. The only people accountable for the decisions and actions taken by readers using the information presented are themselves.

Any names, characters, companies, locations, activities, occasions, and incidents referenced in this book are either made up or the result of the author's imagination. Any likeness to real people, living or dead, or to real things is entirely coincidental.

This book's content may change at any time, without prior notice, according to the author. The onus is on the reader to verify whether there have been any updates or revisions.

The reader accepts the conditions of this disclaimer by reading this book. Please do not read this book or use its contents if you do not agree to these terms.

CHAPTER 1

LEARNING ABOUT VITILIGO

Could you tell me what vitiligo is?

The skin disorder known as vitiligo causes areas of white skin due to the loss of pigment. The loss of function or destruction of the melanocytes—the cells that produce melanin—is the cause of this. Any region of the body is fair game, including the face, hands, and arms.

Vitiligo Causes

Although researchers have not pinpointed a single reason for vitiligo, they do believe that environmental, immunological, and genetic variables all play a role. An important component is autoimmune factors, in which the immune system of the body targets and kills melanocytes by mistake. Because vitiligo is often hereditary, heredity is another factor. Stress, sunburn, or exposure to specific chemicals are also potential causes that might worsen the illness.

Vitiligo Varieties

distinct patterns and levels of pigment loss indicate distinct forms of vitiligo. Some examples are:

1. The majority of cases of vitiligo are non-segmental varieties, which manifest as white spots that are symmetrical on both sides of the body.

2. White patches that are limited to a specific area or side of the body are characteristic of segmental vitiligo, a form of the condition that most commonly affects younger people.

3. In extremely rare instances, vitiligo can spread to almost every part of the body, causing extensive discoloration.

Warning Indicias

White patches, which may start small but gradually become larger over time, appear on the skin as the main symptom of vitiligo. People with darker skin tones tend to notice these areas more. Lips and genitalia aren't the only mucous membranes that can be depigmented by vitiligo.

Identifying Vitiligo

Dermatologists use physical examinations of the skin to diagnose vitiligo. Areas of depigmentation may be brought to light using a Wood's lamp in some instances. To further confirm that the afflicted skin does not contain any melanocytes, a biopsy may be taken.

Atopic Dermatitis and Autoimmune Disorders

Thyroid problems, RA, type 1 diabetes, and vitiligo are autoimmune diseases that frequently occur together. Vitiligo is an autoimmune disorder in which the immune system attacks melanocytes, as it does with other cells and organs.

Hereditary Vitiligo

There is a genetic component to vitiligo, however it is not completely inherited. Vitiligo is more common in people who have a personal or family history of the disorder. The fact that vitiligo does not appear in all people who have a hereditary tendency suggests that additional variables are at play.

Truth and Fiction Around Vitiligo

People often mistakenly believe that vitiligo is caused by poor hygiene or is communicable. Vitiligo is not related to cleanliness and is not communicable. Environmental and genetic factors both have a role in this complicated autoimmune disorder. Some treatments can help control the problem and make the skin look better.

Effects of Vitiligo on Emotional Well-being

Particularly for those who see noticeable changes to their appearance, vitiligo can have a profound effect on mental health, causing feelings of inadequacy, worry, and despair. The psychological effects of vitiligo can be better managed with the use of coping mechanisms such as dermatological treatments, support groups, and therapy.

Children with Vitiligo

Childhood is one of the ages at which vitiligo can manifest. Issues with self-esteem and social interactions may be more difficult for children who have vitiligo. To assist children cope with the psychological and physiological effects of vitiligo, parents and other caretakers must be there for them emotionally and provide them with the medical treatment they need.

In sum, vitiligo can affect one's physical and mental health, and comprehending it requires being aware of all of these factors. To better understand vitiligo, develop effective therapies, and provide support to those living with the illness, healthcare providers, researchers, and people impacted by the condition must work together.

CHAPTER 2

APPROACHES TO TREATMENT

Localised Remedies

The initial step in combating vitiligo is often to apply a topical therapy. Among these, you can find calcineurin inhibitors, vitamin D analogs, and corticosteroids. These drugs aid in repigmentation by reducing the immune response and increasing melanocyte activity in the afflicted regions.

Light therapy (Ultraviolet A and UVB

The process of phototherapy entails exposing the skin to light with a UV wavelength. In contrast to UVB therapy, which just makes use of UVB light, PUVA therapy also makes use of light-sensitizing medicine. Both approaches have the potential to effectively treat extensive vitiligo by increasing melanocyte production.

Endo-Light Laser Treatment

To treat areas of skin discoloration, excimer lasers focus focused UVB light on those areas. Compared to conventional phototherapy, this tailored method for localized vitiligo may be quicker and more successful.

Pills for the Mouth

If your vitiligo is extensive or worsening quickly, your doctor may recommend oral corticosteroids, immunomodulators, or antioxidants. Internally, these drugs modify the immune system and lessen inflammation.

Cosmetic Procedures (Tattooing, Skin Grafting)

In cases where previous therapies have failed to alleviate stable vitiligo, surgical solutions may be explored. Tattooing employs specialized ink to conceal white patches, while skin grafting involves transplanting pigmented skin to depigmented areas.

Investigational Interventions

Novel approaches to treating vitiligo, like as stem cell therapy, melanocyte transplantation, and JAK inhibitors, are the subject of active investigation. The results of these experimental treatments for skin repigmentation are encouraging, suggesting they could eventually enter the mainstream.

Various Treatment Options

To improve results and address several vitiligo symptoms at once, it is recommended to combine different treatment modalities, such as topical medicine with phototherapy or oral medication with surgical treatments.

Natural Curatives and Non-Conventional Medicine

Home remedies, such as topical herbal preparations, dietary adjustments, and stress management strategies, can help alleviate symptoms of vitiligo. However, they should not be relied upon as a replacement for medical therapies. But before you try these methods, talk to your doctor.

Treating Adverse Drug Reactions

Redness, itchiness, or photosensitivity are common side effects of many vitiligo therapies. Oral medicines might also have systemic effects. The key to successfully managing these side effects is close monitoring and open contact with healthcare experts.

Approaches to Treating Vitiligo in the Future

Personalized medicine, tailored medicines, and a better knowledge of the immunological systems involved are the future directions in vitiligo treatment. More precise and personalized treatments may be on the horizon thanks to developments in immunotherapy, gene editing, and biologics.

It is essential to collaborate closely with dermatologists or specialists to create a personalized treatment plan for vitiligo because each patient's experience with the condition and reaction to therapies can differ. For optimal results, it may be necessary to conduct regular follow-ups and make modifications.

CHAPTER 3

MANAGING YOUR LIFESTYLE

Tips for Vitiligo Skincare: Taking good care of one's skin is an important part of dealing with vitiligo. Dry, flaky skin can make vitiligo spots look even worse, therefore it's important to keep your skin moisturized. To keep irritation at bay, choose mild, fragrance-free moisturizers. Another technique to keep skin healthy without removing its natural oils is to use a gentle cleanser. Because sun exposure can cause vitiligo patches to appear or worsen, it is important to regularly apply sunscreen to safeguard affected regions.

Sunscreens and Protective Clothing:

People with vitiligo must take extra precautions to avoid sun exposure. Excessive time in the sun can cause sunburn and subsequent skin discoloration. To protect oneself from both UVA and UVB radiation, it is recommended to wear broad-spectrum sunscreens with an SPF of 30 or higher. Remember to reapply it after swimming or perspiring. Further advice: stay out of the sun during its hottest hours and use protective gear like caps and long sleeves.

How to Use Makeup to Hide Vitiligo:

If you suffer from vitiligo, you can hide the spots and feel more self-confident by using makeup. Pick hypoallergenic, high-quality items that complement the skin tone. To reduce the visual difference between areas of pigmentation and those without, try using a concealer or color-correcting lotion. Carefully blend for a natural look, and if you want personalized recommendations, consider seeing a makeup professional who has expertise working with vitiligo patients.

Tips for Managing Vitiligo through Fashion and Clothing Choices:

Choosing your clothes carefully can help. If you want to hide depigmented spots, try wearing dark-colored clothing. Patterns and textures can also help. Cotton and other lightweight, breathable textiles are soft and pleasant to the skin. Inspire the person to try on a variety of looks until they discover one that suits them.

Counseling and psychological support:

vitiligo can greatly affect mental health. Patients greatly benefit from counseling and psychological support when navigating their emotions and self-image. Prompt them to look into support groups or professional counseling so they may talk to others going through the same things, learn how to cope, and become more resilient.

Many people with vitiligo find that they need time to work on their self-confidence. Promote healthy habits of self-care and positive self-talk. Put less emphasis on outward looks and more on inside qualities and accomplishments. Participating in things that make you happy and fulfilled can also improve your self-esteem and general health.

A healthy, well-balanced diet promotes skin health in general, and while no one diet will cure vitiligo, it can help. Insist that people eat plenty of fresh produce, lean meats, and healthy fats. Vitamin D and B12 supplements are an option for some people, but before making any major changes to their diet, it is important to talk to their doctor.

Regular exercise has several positive effects on vitiligo patients, including elevating their mood and improving blood flow. Strive for a balanced workout routine that includes cardio, strength training, and stretching. Sun protection should be worn in conjunction with outdoor activities. A healthy outlet for stress management is exercise.

Dealing with Stress:

Managing stress is crucial for general health, particularly for people dealing with long-term disorders like vitiligo. Promote relaxation techniques like yoga, deep breathing, meditation, or enjoyable pastimes. Another way to reduce stress is to set reasonable goals and boundaries and to ask for help when you need it.

Relationship and Social Interaction Management:

Living with vitiligo can make it difficult to manage relationships and social interactions. To promote understanding and support, encourage loved ones to talk openly about the disease. It might also be helpful in social situations to address misconceptions regarding vitiligo. Inspire people to take part in group outings that foster acceptance and positivity.

Overall, people with vitiligo can empower themselves to live full lives with resilience and confidence with a comprehensive approach that includes skincare, sun protection, cosmetics methods, psychological support, self-care practices, good lifestyle choices, and positive social interactions.

CHAPTER 4

FACING VITILIGO EVERY DAY

Maintenance Schedules:

To keep vitiligo under control, it is necessary to adhere to a daily maintenance regimen. Things like:

1. To maintain healthy skin and prevent irritation, it is vital to cleanse gently with fragrance-free, gentle solutions. It is especially vital to moisturize regions affected by vitiligo frequently to keep the skin hydrated.

2. Sunscreen with a high SPF and protective gear are essential for vitiligo patients to avoid further skin discoloration caused by sunburn.

3. To hide the appearance of uneven pigmentation, some people use self-tanners or cosmetic makeup. Hypoallergenic and non-comedogenic products should be used.

4. Mental health care is just as vital as physical health care for emotional wellness. To alleviate the emotional toll that vitiligo takes, try mindfulness practices, reach out to friends and family for support, or see a therapist.

Aspects of Your Job and Your Future:

Here are some things to think about if you have vitiligo and are pursuing a career:

1. Building self-confidence is essential for vitiligo employees. One way to combat prejudice and discrimination is to highlight your strengths.

2. It is a personal decision whether to tell your employer or coworkers about your vitiligo. It can help to know your rights under laws that pertain to people with disabilities.

3. Workplace accommodations: If vitiligo gets in the way of your job, talk to your boss about ways you may work around it, like asking for more

leeway in your schedule or asking for ergonomic modifications.

When veils are involved:

Some preparation is required when traveling with vitiligo:

1. Sunscreen, caps, and UV-protective clothes should be in your travel kit to keep the sun's rays at bay.

2. Take with you any oral or topical drugs you take regularly, as well as any relevant doctor's notes.

3. Makeup and concealment: Bring enough of your favorite cosmetics to last the whole vacation.

The Risk of Vitiligo During Pregnancy:

While vitiligo usually doesn't interfere with pregnancy, the hormonal changes that occur during the process can:

1. For individualized advice on how to deal with vitiligo while pregnant, see your obstetrician and dermatologist.

2. Pregnancy hormones can make skin more sensitive, so it's important to prioritize sun protection and stick to a gentle skincare routine.

Age-Related Vitiligo:

Certain difficulties may arise for people with vitiligo as they get older:

1. Age-Related Skin Changes: Sun protection and frequent moisturization are crucial as we age because our skin may become more dry and thinner.

2. Cosmetic Issues: If you're self-conscious about changes in your pigmentation patterns or the difference between your pigmented and depigmented areas, there are cosmetic options available to you.

Support and Advocacy Organisations:

Joining an advocacy group or finding a support network can help you get the information and emotional assistance you need:

1. Get the word out about vitiligo advocacy and support groups that host events, forums, and informational resources for the community.

2. Empowerment: Take part in campaigns to get the word out, encourage research, and fight for tolerance and inclusion.

Motivational Tales from Those Fighting Vitiligo:

It is possible to spread optimism and support by sharing the stories of people who have overcome vitiligo:

1. Community Forums: Speak out about your experiences with vitiligo on social media, via blogs, or at public speaking events to encourage others.

2. Encourage self-determination among people living with vitiligo by showcasing their strengths, accomplishments, and constructive coping mechanisms.

Famous people with vitiligo include:

Famous people who have vitiligo might be great inspirations:

1. Notoriety: When famous people talk about their vitiligo experiences, it raises awareness and acceptance.

2. Their prominence in the entertainment and media industries helps to promote diversity and inclusion.

Creative Expression of Vitiligo: Art and Creativity

People who have vitiligo may find that creative expression helps:

1. Tattoos and other forms of body art allow some people to creatively express and revel in their distinct skin patterns.

2. Projects in photography and the visual arts that feature vitiligo have the potential to educate the public and urge them to reevaluate conventional notions of beauty.

Fight Intolerance and Misconduct:

Advocacy and education are necessary to fight prejudice and stigma:

1. Raising Awareness: Spread the word about vitiligo, its causes, and why inclusivity and acceptance are so important.

2. Protest: Rally around causes and programs that expand access to quality healthcare, quality education, and inclusive workplaces.

Dealing with vitiligo requires a multi-pronged strategy that includes skincare, mental health, activism, and embracing variety and innovation. Everyone may live a full life and make a good impact when people with vitiligo receive the care, support, and information they need.

CHAPTER 5

INVESTIGATIONS AND PROGRESS

Latest Findings in Vitiligo Research

Loss of pigment-producing cells causes depigmented areas on the skin in the complicated skin disease vitiligo. Understanding the etiology of vitiligo, creating effective treatments, and enhancing the quality of life for affected persons are the current foci of multi-domain research.

Vitiligo: A Genetic and Immunological Study

The immunological and genetic components of vitiligo have recently become the subject of much research. The genetic components of the disease have been better-understood thanks to the identification of many susceptibility loci. From an immunological perspective, our knowledge of how vitiligo develops is expanding; specifically, how immune cells attack melanocytes and cause pigment loss is becoming clearer.

Novel Therapeutic Approaches and Clinical Trials

New treatments for vitiligo must undergo rigorous testing in clinical trials. Newer studies have investigated immunomodulatory drugs, phototherapy regimens adapted to each patient's unique profile, and JAK inhibitors, among other innovative treatments. Emerging treatments are guided by the data provided by these trials, which offer significant information on efficacy, safety, and long-term consequences.

Medical Regenerative Science and Stem Cell Treatment

By restoring damaged melanocytes, stem cell therapy has potential as a treatment for vitiligo. To replenish pigment cells in areas that have lost their pigmentation, scientists are looking into several stem cell sources, such as induced pluripotent stem cells and autologous melanocyte transplantation. Restoring skin pigmentation and stopping the course of illness are the goals of regenerative therapies.

Technologies in Genomic Engineering and CRISPR

New opportunities have arisen in the study of vitiligo thanks to developments in CRISPR and genetic engineering. To treat vitiligo and other hereditary disorders as well as to alter immune responses that target melanocytes, researchers are investigating gene editing approaches. Potentially individualized treatments based on genetic profiles are within reach with the help of these state-of-the-art technologies.

Potential Biomarkers for the Tracking of Vitiligo Development

Research is mostly focused on identifying biomarkers that indicate the progression of vitiligo. Genetic markers, cytokine levels, and profiles of particular immune cells are all examples of biomarkers that can be used to forecast the course of a disease, its prognosis, and the efficacy of a treatment. Precision medicine methods for vitiligo management are enhanced by integrating biomarker data into clinical treatment.

Worldwide Efforts to Raise Awareness of Vitiligo

The goals of these worldwide campaigns are to educate the public about vitiligo, dispel myths about the condition, and push for more equitable healthcare policy. Worldwide, groups like the Vitiligo Research Foundation (VRF) and World Vitiligo Day (WVD) work to raise awareness, funds for research, and community support for vitiligo patients. Researchers, physicians, and advocacy groups work together more effectively through these projects.

Joint Work by Patients and Scientists

To improve patient outcomes and advance vitiligo research, patient-researcher collaborations are crucial. Individuals living with vitiligo are empowered to have a say in research goals, clinical trial design, and therapy development through patient-centered research initiatives. These initiatives include patient advocacy groups, support networks, and participatory research methods.

Comprehensive Methods for Studying Vitiligo

Vitiligo research that takes a holistic approach draws from a variety of fields to examine the condition from every angle, including the physical, psychological, social, and quality of life dimensions. Comprehensive care models that address the holistic requirements of individuals with vitiligo, including mental health assistance and societal engagement, are achieved through the integration of dermatology, immunology, psychology, and social sciences.

The Way Forward for Vitiligo Studies

Personalized treatments based on genetic profiling, immune modulation tactics, and advances in regenerative medicine are just a few of the fascinating prospects for vitiligo research in the future. The complicated nature of vitiligo will only be better understood and treated via multidisciplinary collaboration, worldwide awareness campaigns, and patient-centered initiatives.

CHAPTER 6

JUVENILE VITILIGO

How Vitiligo Emerges in Childhood

A skin disorder known as vitiligo causes areas of white skin caused by the loss of skin pigment. Vitiligo can strike at any age, even youngsters, but there are special precautions when it first appears in children. Vitiligo usually doesn't show up until a person is at least 20 years old, though it can happen as early as birth in rare instances. A mix of hereditary, autoimmune, and environmental variables contribute to the complicated and poorly understood etiology of vitiligo.

Effects on Families and Children

Beyond the obvious skin discoloration, vitiligo has far-reaching effects on affected children and their families. Bullying, low self-esteem, and negative cultural views can all contribute to emotional suffering in children. Medical treatments, societal stigma, and emotional support for children can all be difficult for families to manage.

Strategies for the Treatment of Children

Repigmentation of afflicted regions and management of symptoms are the main goals of treatment for pediatric vitiligo. Possible treatments include phototherapy, calcineurin inhibitors, topical corticosteroids, and even surgical procedures such as skin grafting or melanocyte transplantation. Treatment options are determined by the severity of vitiligo, the age of the child, and their general health.

Obstacles in the Classroom and Life

Due to misunderstandings regarding their disease, children with vitiligo may have difficulties in social and educational contexts. Teaching others about vitiligo can help break down prejudice and increase acceptance. Children can learn to accept and value themselves more when adults encourage open conversation and provide a nurturing atmosphere.

Resources and Assistance Tailored to Children

Children and their families dealing with vitiligo can benefit greatly from child-friendly materials including books, films, and online groups. Kids can learn more about their illness, make friends with others who understand, and develop resilience with the help of these tools.

Advice for the Caretakers and Parents

When it comes to helping children who have vitiligo, parents and carers are invaluable. Some suggestions include parents learning more about the disease, encouraging open communication, standing up for their child's needs, encouraging positive body image and self-esteem, and reaching out to healthcare providers and support groups for assistance.

Championing the Cause of Vitiligo in Children

Children with vitiligo have an advocate who works to get the word out, encourage acceptance, and secure resources for those who suffer from the condition. Children with vitiligo have advocates who fight to dispel myths, end discrimination, and foster acceptance and understanding.

Children with Vitiligo Need Positive Adult Role Models

Celebrities or community leaders who have vitiligo can serve as positive role models for children, showing them that their condition does not limit their potential or value. By overcoming obstacles and embracing their individuality, these role models can help children succeed.

School-Based Educational Programmes

Schools can take action to make their communities more accepting of students who have vitiligo by implementing educational activities. Awareness campaigns, diversity training for teachers and students, and policies that encourage inclusion and tolerance for children who have apparent differences are all examples of what can fall under this category of projects.

Fostering Resilience in Youth With Vitiligo

Confidence, coping mechanisms, a positive self-image, and emotional support are all important components of a resilient adolescent vitiligo patient. Children with vitiligo can flourish despite the difficulties they face if they participate in resilience-building activities, attend peer support groups, and undergo cognitive-behavioral treatment.

Children with vitiligo can be better supported by healthcare providers, schools, families, and communities if these factors are addressed holistically. This will enable these children to lead confident and fulfilled lives.

CHAPTER 7

VITILIGO AND EMOTIONAL WELL-BEING

Effects of Vitiligo on the Mind

The psychological toll of vitiligo, a disorder defined by a gradual or sudden loss of skin pigmentation, can be substantial. Feelings of inadequacy, low self-esteem, and, in extreme circumstances, despair or worry might result from the condition's obvious visibility. To effectively manage vitiligo, it is vital to cope with these psychological obstacles.

Coping Mechanisms for Mental Anxiety

People with vitiligo can find relief from the emotional distress it causes by employing one of several coping mechanisms. Some of these strategies include learning to reframe negative views about one's looks, taking care of oneself, doing things that make one happy and fulfilled, reaching out to loved ones for support, and so on.

Counseling and Therapy Alternatives

For those dealing with the emotional toll that vitiligo takes, therapy and counseling can be life-changing. For instance, cognitive-behavioral therapy (CBT) can assist people in identifying and altering unhelpful ways of thinking as well as in constructing more adaptive strategies for dealing with stressful situations.

Ways to Practice Mindfulness and Meditation

Practicing mindfulness and meditation can also aid in stress management and general well-being. By engaging in these activities, people with chronic conditions can learn to manage their anxiety, focus on the here and now, and practice self-compassion.

Enhancing Confidence and Embracing One's Body

Individuals with vitiligo must prioritize their mental health by building self-esteem and promoting body positivity. Some ways to achieve this goal include building relationships that support and validate you, focusing on your strengths, and learning to accept yourself as you are.

Group Therapy and Adolescent Mentoring

People with vitiligo might find a sense of community and acceptance through peer counseling or support groups. Making connections with people who understand what you're going through might help you feel less alone and provide much-needed emotional support.

Coping with Depression and Anxiety

Treatment for vitiligo-related anxiety and depression may involve talk therapy, medication (if needed), and behavioral adjustments. If people are dealing with ongoing emotions of sadness or worry, they must get assistance from a mental health expert.

Struggling with Social Isolation

For people who experience stigmatisation or miscommunication because of their vitiligo, social isolation can be a formidable obstacle. One strategy to fight social isolation is to find ways to connect with other people. This can be done through online communities, support groups, or social events.

Promoting Mental Health Through Empowerment

To combat stigma, increase understanding, and promote easily available mental health services, it is essential to strengthen the voice of the vitiligo community's mental health advocates. Those who are willing to stand up and share their stories can help bring about change.

Approaching Vitiligo from a Holistic Perspective

People with vitiligo can benefit from holistic wellness measures that include things like eating healthily, exercising regularly, getting enough sleep, and learning to handle stress. It is possible to improve one's physical and mental health by adopting a holistic approach to wellness.

Therapy, self-care routines, social support, and advocacy activities are all part of the complex puzzle when it comes to vitiligo's psychological impact. It is possible to live a full life despite vitiligo if one puts their mental health and well-being first.

CHAPTER 8

VITILIGO AND EMOTIONAL WELL-BEING

Effects of Vitiligo on the Mind

Vitiligo affects more than just the skin; it can have a major influence on a person's mental health as well. Feelings of shame, insecurity, and poor self-esteem may accompany the abrupt emergence of white patches on the skin. Anxieties, sadness, and social isolation are common among vitiligo patients because they are constantly worried about how others will see them.

Coping Mechanisms for Mental Anxiety

Developing appropriate coping mechanisms is essential for managing the emotional suffering associated with vitiligo. Some ways to do this include talking to people you care about, doing things that make you happy, taking care of yourself, and changing the way you think about criticisms of your looks. One way to deal with the emotional difficulties of vitiligo is to work on building resilience and a positive attitude.

Counseling and Therapy Alternatives

For those dealing with the emotional toll that vitiligo takes, therapy and counseling can be life-changing. Improving coping mechanisms and addressing negative thought patterns are two goals of cognitive-behavioral therapy (CBT). Psychotherapy also offers a secure environment where one can learn to cope with stressful and anxious feelings by examining their thoughts and feelings.

Ways to Practice Mindfulness and Meditation

Reducing stress and enhancing overall well-being can be achieved through mindfulness and meditation activities. These methods include accepting oneself as one is, regardless of how one seems on the outside, practicing self-compassion, and living in the now. People who suffer from vitiligo might find a sense of stability and strength by practicing mindfulness in their everyday lives.

Enhancing Confidence and Embracing One's Body

Important parts of dealing with the mental effects of vitiligo include boosting self-esteem and encouraging body positivity. Some ways to achieve this goal include questioning conventional ideas of beauty, celebrating differences, and putting more emphasis on character traits than on physical attributes. Boosting self-esteem can also be achieved by surrounding oneself with supportive communities and engaging in positive affirmations.

Group Therapy and Adolescent Mentoring

People with vitiligo can find emotional support and validation through peer counseling and support groups. Reducing feelings of loneliness and increasing acceptance can be achieved through connecting with others who share similar experiences. The ability to learn from one another's experiences and share coping mechanisms is a key component of peer counseling.

Coping with Depression and Anxiety

People who suffer from vitiligo often struggle with mental health issues like anxiety and sadness. If these symptoms continue or become a problem for you to deal with regularly, it is crucial to consult a doctor. Modifying one's lifestyle to include things like getting enough sleep, eating well, and exercising regularly can help with anxiety and depression management, in addition to treatment.

Struggling with Social Isolation

A major worry for those with obvious differences, such as vitiligo, is the possibility of social isolation. If you suffer from feelings of loneliness or isolation, it may help to find ways to interact with other people. This could be through online communities, social activities, or support groups. One of the most effective ways to combat feelings of loneliness is to cultivate genuine connections with people via compassion and understanding.

Promoting Mental Health Through Empowerment

Bringing attention to the emotional toll of vitiligo and fighting for more welcoming policies and resources is an important part of empowering mental health activism. People with vitiligo may help build a more accepting and inclusive society by speaking up about their experiences, fighting stigma, and advocating for diversity and inclusion.

Approaching Vitiligo from a Holistic Perspective

Caring for one's mind, body, and soul is a holistic approach to wellness for vitiligo patients. Among these include making mental and physical well-being a priority through self-care routines, maintaining a healthy weight, regularly exercising, and engaging in stress-reducing activities like yoga and tai chi. Effective management of vitiligo requires a holistic approach that acknowledges the interdependence of physical and mental health.

Through the implementation of proactive coping mechanisms, therapy, support networks, and holistic health practices, individuals can improve their quality of life and develop resilience when dealing with the psychological effects of vitiligo.

CHAPTER 9

COMMON QUESTIONS AND ADVICE FROM INDUSTRY PROFESSIONALS IN

Vitiligo: Frequently Asked Questions:

1. Vitiligo, what is it? A skin disorder known as vitiligo causes patches of white skin to appear where color has been lost.

2. How does vitiligo develop? Although researchers have not pinpointed a single cause, they suspect that environmental, autoimmune, and genetic variables all have a role.

3. How infectious is vitiligo? Having vitiligo does not make you infectious. This condition cannot be transmitted to others.

4. Will vitiligo ever fade away? There may not be a cure for vitiligo, but there are therapies that can

help with management and even out the skin's look.

5. Is vitiligo so common? Vitiligo is a skin disorder that affects approximately 1-2 percent of the world's population. It affects people of both sexes and all races.

Recommendations from Industry Experts:

For further information about vitiligo management tactics, treatment choices, and the most recent studies, consult a dermatologist or specialist.

Discussions with Skin Specialists:

The diagnosis, treatment, and continued care of vitiligo patients can be better understood by speaking with dermatologists. New treatments can be discussed, and they can offer advice on how to manage the illness.

New Information from Vitiligo Experts:

Scientists who study vitiligo can keep us informed of new findings regarding the condition, its causes, and possible therapies. Their findings may provide optimism for the development of new treatments for vitiligo.

Feedback & Accounts from Patients:

Having the opportunity to hear from others who are vitiligo survivors can be helpful, both emotionally and practically. People with vitiligo can find strength in one another's experiences, and their stories can serve as an inspiration to others.

Advice from Experts on Vitiligo:

Experts in vitiligo treatment can provide helpful advice on how to cope with symptoms, pick out clothes and sunscreen that will accentuate your condition, and feel comfortable in social settings.

Dispelling Vitiligo Myths:

Many people have the wrong idea about vitiligo, thinking it's communicable or uncurable. Education and awareness campaigns dispelling these stereotypes can aid in the fight against stigma and for better understanding.

Dealing with Divisive Subjects:

Discussions on experimental treatments, cultural views of the disorder, and obstacles patients encounter in obtaining adequate care are all potential sources of controversy in vitiligo therapy.

Outlook for Vitiligo Treatment in the Future:

The future of vitiligo care, according to experts, could bring new treatments, a better understanding of the disease's processes, and better patient support services.

Regular dermatological appointments, treatment plan adherence, and emotional well-being management are all examples of practical guidance that experts can give patients. Help for carers dealing with vitiligo is also available.

Individuals can improve their knowledge of vitiligo, its treatment, and available resources by attending to these details thoroughly.

CHAPTER 10

SUPPORTING AND ENCOURAGING

Supporting Patients with Vitiligo

Patients with vitiligo can empower themselves by learning about their illness, coping with emotional difficulties, and taking charge of their healing process. It includes teaching people about the illness and all they can do to get better, such as what causes it and how to treat it. To manage the emotional and social effects of vitiligo, it is important to empower people by boosting their self-esteem, confidence, and resilience.

Capacity for Self-Advocacy

Patients with vitiligo must learn to advocate for themselves to get the help they need. Participation in treatment decisions requires open and honest communication with healthcare providers, including the expression of concerns, questions, and answers. Seeking out knowledge, support groups, and resources to empower oneself and make educated choices is also part of self-advocacy.

Bringing Attention to Neighbourhoods

To fight stigma, increase understanding, and foster acceptance, it is crucial to raise community knowledge about vitiligo. Public awareness efforts, media relations, social media campaigns, and other similar endeavors can accomplish this. As part of this, individuals with vitiligo should share their stories, debunk misconceptions, and bring attention to the variety of experiences that this condition can cause.

Supporting a Diverse and Inclusive Environment

The best way to encourage diversity and inclusion is to make sure that everyone feels welcome and valued, regardless of their background or identity. It entails fighting for vitiligo-inclusive policy, media and advertising representation, and equal opportunity for those with the condition.

Joining Clinical Trials and Other Research Projects

If we want to learn more about vitiligo, develop better treatments, and ultimately find a cure, we must participate in research and clinical trials. One way to be involved is to volunteer for studies, which allows you to have a say in what studies are prioritized. Another way is to lobby for more money and support for vitiligo research.

Interacting with the Public and Media

Vitiligo sufferers can help dispel myths and spread awareness by taking part in public discourse and sharing their own experiences through various media outlets. Accurate and sympathetic media coverage of vitiligo is a goal that can be achieved by collaboration with news outlets, bloggers, influencers, and advocacy groups.

Aiding Groups Focused on Vitiligo

The community, advocacy, and helpful resources provided by vitiligo organizations are invaluable to patients and their families. Volunteering, fundraising, attending events, and spreading the word about these organizations' work to help vitiligo patients are all part of it.

Championing Healthcare Rights in Legislation

Access to healthcare, insurance coverage, and financing for vitiligo research are all areas that can be influenced through legislative campaigning. It entails coordinating with lawmakers, pushing for appropriate legislation, and defending the healthcare system's treatment of vitiligo sufferers.

Honoring the Pride of Vitiligo

Taking pleasure in vitiligo means accepting one's individuality, encouraging self-acceptance, and questioning conventional notions of beauty. To help individuals with vitiligo feel confident in their skin and empowered by their condition, it is important to host events, spread encouraging words online, and build a community of support.

Promoting Embracing Change

A cultural movement towards appreciating diversity, combating stereotypes, and cultivating tolerance is essential for inspiring change and acceptance. It entails spreading awareness about vitiligo, encouraging compassion and understanding, and fighting for structural reforms that make everyone feel welcome and valued, no matter how they look.

In conclusion, there is a vast array of endeavors that go under the umbrella of "vitiligo empowerment and advocacy" that seek to enhance results, increase understanding, foster acceptance, and fight for the rights and welfare of vitiligo patients. It calls for teamwork, knowledge, perseverance, and a resolve to build a society that welcomes and supports all people.